ADVANCE PRAISE

"Paul Zak's The Little Book of Happiness delivers a roadmap for deeper joy and meaning, weaving together cutting-edge neuroscience and timeless principles. You will be carrying this in your pocket for years to come."
—DR. ARTHUR C. BROOKS, HARVARD PROFESSOR AND #1 NEW YORK TIMES BESTSELLING AUTHOR

"Paul Zak keeps coming up with amazing insights that enhance our humanity. In this book he shows us a path toward a happy, meaningful life. Learn to live each day with love, compassion, and courage. Learn to follow a life of virtue and joy."
—DR. JOHN GOTTMAN, AUTHOR OF FIGHT RIGHT

"Paul Zak is a master distiller who offers a highly concentrated prescription for happiness. Take two drops and feel happier in the morning!"
—NEIL PASRICHA, AUTHOR OF THE BOOK OF AWESOME: SNOW DAYS, BAKERY AIR, FINDING MONEY IN YOUR POCKET, AND OTHER SIMPLE, BRILLIANT THINGS

"Amid a sea of books promising routes to happiness, The Little Book of Happiness actually delivers. With his deep knowledge of the human brain, backed by decades of scholarly research, Zak provides the reader the conceptual tools—and the app to go with it—to travel on a successful route to that destination we all seek, true happiness."

—DR. ROB KURZBAN, AUTHOR OF WHY EVERYONE (ELSE) IS A HYPOCRITE

"Our brains are naturally lazy, resisting change even when it's for our own good. But with the help of your smartwatch, a unique app, and the actionable insights in this book, you'll learn how to outsmart your brain and build habits that improve your mood, engagement, and overall quality of life."

—DR. MICHAEL WINTERDAHL, ASSOCIATE PROFESSOR AT AALBORG UNIVERSITY

"The Little Book of Happiness is a masterful synthesis of cutting-edge science and practical wisdom. This isn't just another guide to happiness—it's a tool kit for flourishing, backed by neuroscience and decades of research. With his characteristic warmth and clarity, Paul Zak unpacks the role of virtues in building deeper connections and a more fulfilling life. The technology that accompanies the book makes age-old practices actionable for today's world, empowering the cultivation of joy in ways that are both measurable and deeply personal."

—DR. MIKE RUCKER, AUTHOR OF THE FUN HABIT

"The Little Book of Happiness will inspire you with neuroscience and uplift you with virtuous visions. Much more, it will give you a way to measure results in yourself, now. If you want more than talk, this book is for you."

—DR. VANCE Z. JOHNSON, MEDICAL DIRECTOR AT LOMA LINDA UNIVERSITY MEDICAL CENTER

"A great resource on the virtues that will pave your way to happiness—with pragmatic recommendations to help you actually make happiness happen. You won't want to miss this substance-packed little book."

—DR. TRACY BROWER, AUTHOR OF *THE SECRETS TO HAPPINESS AT WORK: HOW TO CHOOSE AND CREATE PURPOSE AND FULFILLMENT IN YOUR WORK*

"Paul's book offers many easy-to-adopt practices that help us experience happiness and grow our joy muscles. Change is hard, especially making lifestyle changes that stick, so it is wonderful that readers can use the SIX app to understand what experiences on any given day are actually increasing their feeling of happiness."

—ANDREW CANNON, FOUNDER OF THE ART AND SCIENCE OF JOY

"Happiness isn't just something that happens to you—it's something you create. In The Little Book of Happiness, Dr. Paul J. Zak shows how small, deliberate choices can transform your mood, relationships, and life. With clear steps and tools like the SIX app, this book enables anyone to build a happier, more meaningful life."

—DAAN VAN ROSSUM, FOUNDER OF FLEXOS

THE LITTLE BOOK OF HAPPINESS

THE
LITTLE BOOK OF
HAPPINESS

A SCIENTIFIC APPROACH TO LIVING BETTER

PAUL J. ZAK

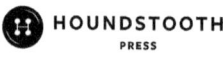
HOUNDSTOOTH
PRESS

COPYRIGHT © 2025 PAUL J. ZAK
All rights reserved.

THE LITTLE BOOK OF HAPPINESS
A Scientific Approach to Living Better

FIRST EDITION

ISBN 978-1-5445-4788-6 *Hardcover*
      978-1-5445-4787-9 *Paperback*
      978-1-5445-4789-3 *Ebook*
      978-1-5445-4790-9 *Audiobook*

To Chris Rufer, a resolute champion of liberty and the pursuit of happiness. The technology to measure happiness upon which this book is based would not be possible without your encouragement, friendship, and support.

CONTENTS

	INTRODUCTION	13
1.	ADAPTABILITY	22
2.	ATTENTION	24
3.	AWE	26
4.	CAUTION	28
5.	COMPASSION	30
6.	COURAGE	32
7.	CREATIVITY	34
8.	CURIOSITY	36
9.	DEFIANCE	38
10.	DEVOTION	40
11.	FAIRNESS	42
12.	FORGIVENESS	44
13.	GENEROSITY	46
14.	GRATITUDE	48
15.	HONESTY	50
16.	HUMOR	52
17.	IMPARTIALITY	54
18.	INDUSTRIOUSNESS	56
19.	INNOCENCE	58
20.	JUSTICE	60
21.	LOVE	62
22.	LOYALTY	64
23.	MAJESTY	66

24. MODERATION	68
25. MODESTY	70
26. OBEDIENCE	72
27. OPENNESS	74
28. PATIENCE	76
29. PATRIOTISM	78
30. PERSEVERANCE	80
31. PRUDENCE	82
32. PURPOSE	84
33. RESPONSIBILITY	86
34. SELF-REGULATION	88
35. SENSITIVITY	90
36. SERENITY	92
37. SILENCE	94
38. SINCERITY	96
39. SPONTANEITY	98
40. TEAMWORK	100
41. TOLERANCE	102
42. TOUGHNESS	104
43. TRUST	106
44. TRUSTWORTHINESS	108
45. WISDOM	110
CONCLUSION	113

INTRODUCTION

Benjamin Franklin was a most practical thinker. He flew a kite with a key attached not because he was interested in the physical properties of electricity, but because he wanted to improve people's lives. In 1749 he wrote that he was "chagrin'd a little" that his studies of electricity had produced "Nothing in this Way of Use to Mankind." His experiments led to Franklin's invention of the lightning rod, which did help mankind. He also successfully cooked turkeys with electricity, reporting that "the birds kill'd in this manner eat uncommonly tender."

Franklin was a voracious reader and was interested in self-improvement. He had supported himself since he was seventeen years old, and his successes were due in large part to taking risks and learning new skills. One of the books Franklin read was by the classical Greek philosopher Aristotle. Aristotle proposed that a person who was virtuous would achieve *eudaimonia*, or flourishing. In other words, by making a habit of virtues, one would live a happy and fulfilled life.

But how does one practice virtues, and which ones?

Franklin read some more and came up with twelve virtues. He then made a chart of these virtues and a box for each day so he could check them off to help him form habits so that the virtues were second nature.

Franklin met monthly with a group of men he called his "junto," with whom he exchanged ideas for mutual improvement. Franklin was excited to share with the junto members his discovery of twelve virtues and the system he had created to become happier. After his presentation, one member, a Quaker medical doctor, pulled Ben aside and told him that his "pride showed itself frequently in conversation; that [he] was not content with being in the right when discussing any point but was overbearing and rather insolent."[1] Franklin took this critique to heart and added a thirteenth virtue: humility. Later in life, Franklin believed it was his humility that increased his "influence in public councils when [he] became a member."

Franklin was not the only revolutionary leader of the breakaway colonies to embrace virtue for self-improvement. When George Washington was sixteen years old, he copied a list of 110 "Rules of Civility and Decent Behavior in Company and Conversation" from a book put together in 1595 by French Jesuit priests.[2] Washington copied and reviewed these rules to shape his behavior and build a strong moral core that served him well as a leader.

---

[1] Franklin autobiography, quoted in https://thefederalist.com/2021/05/13/what-benjamin-franklins-autobiography-can-teach-us-about-humility/.

[2] George Washington, George Washington: A Collection, compiled and edited by W.B. Allen (Indianapolis: Liberty Fund, 1988), Chapter: Chronology Accessed from http://oll.libertyfund.org/title/848/101681.

Today it is generally accepted that there are forty-five cardinal virtues; each of these is included in this book. Decades of research in neuroscience and positive psychology have confirmed Aristotle's assertion that virtuous behaviors improve the quality of life. They do this because virtuous behaviors are "prosocial." That means they put others ahead of oneself and in doing so draw others to us.

Research by Oxford University has shown that about one-half of our happiness can be traced to having a rich social network. There is no question that as social creatures, social connections are essential for us to thrive. Indeed, having a close group of people who truly care about you is more effective at extending healthspan than is quitting smoking. Put another way, a large study reported a 50 percent increase in the likelihood of survival at every age for those with strong social relationships compared to those without them.[3] The anatomy of the human brain reveals that we are truly a social species: we have hypertrophied brain regions that process social-emotional information compared to our nonhuman primate cousins.

Since everyone wants to be happier, the key question is: what does having a "rich" social network mean exactly? The number of friends on your phone contact list? The number of people you talk to in a day? And, importantly, how does one add to the richness of one's social network?

---

[3] Julianne Holt-Lunstad, Timothy B. Smith, and J. Bradley Layton, "Social Relationships and Mortality Risk: A Meta-analytic Review," PLoS Med 7, no. 7 (2010), https://doi.org/10.1371/journal.pmed.1000316.

There are two answers to these questions. The first is that we can enrich our social networks by investing in relationships. My published scientific research shows that people who consistently invest in serving others have exceptionally strong brain activity supporting social connections. As a result, they have closer relationships with friends, parents, spouses, and work colleagues. These prosocial investments have enriched their social networks, and the data shows that these super-connectors are happier and live longer. They practice many of the virtues Ben Franklin codified.

Here is the science: the brain is constantly adapting to our internal and external environments, and by following the program in this book you can strengthen the social-connection network in your brain and realize the benefits of a rich social network. You will become a super-connector.

The second part of the happiness-improvement program is measurement. This book comes with a free app that continuously measures the neurologic value of the experiences you have. Prosocial behaviors excite the brain's social-emotional valuation network. Consistently spiking this network causes the brain to default to prosociality, increasing the quality of social connections and thereby happiness. As you follow Franklin and practice the virtues—that is, practice being prosocial—the free app that comes with this book will show you objectively just how much happier you are. No journaling, no letter-writing. Rather, you will get an objective measurement of the value your brain obtains from prosocial behaviors. The app also provides clear goals that will guide you to greater flourishing.

Like all important endeavors, it will take some work. But the goal is easy: six.

Peer-reviewed research from my lab shows that to increase happiness, you need to have six high-value experiences a day. Your goal is six and the free app, of course called SIX, will show which experiences are the most neurologically valuable to you. My peer-reviewed research shows that these high-value experiences boost one's mood and energy.

The SIX app captures the activity of two neurochemicals that the brain uses to value social-emotional experiences: dopamine and oxytocin. These neurochemicals induce electrical activity that is sent through the brain's "output file," the cranial nerves, from the brain to the body. Over many years, my team traced the pathways from the brain's social-emotional valuation network to the cranial nerves and then wrote algorithms that enable us to measure the value of experiences in real time. The SIX app does this by applying algorithms to signals we pull from fitness wearables and smartwatches. The "magic" of this technology is that some of the cranial nerves innervate the heart, and we showed that dopamine and oxytocin subtly affect cardiac rhythms that our algorithms capture. To be clear, SIX does not measure your heart rate or heart rate variability as these do not predict happiness-improving behaviors. Rather, SIX captures very subtle changes in the control of cardiac responses that we identified by pharmacologically manipulating dopamine and oxytocin.

Consistently reaching six key moments a day, as shown using SIX, not only increases happiness, but will improve your long-term satisfaction with life. This is why you should try to complete the practices in all chapters in this book.

Step one on your happiness journey is to download the SIX app by scanning this QR code.

Measure yourself today before getting too far into the book to baseline your thriving. People who have zero to three peak value moments a day tend to have low energy and low mood. If that is you, do not worry. The set of exercises in this book, if practiced, will improve this number. And, more is better. Readers who already have strong social connections may have ten or twelve high-value experiences on some days. Bravo! Keep connecting and keep following the practices in this book to get even happier.

As you become proficient in the prosocial virtues, the number of key moments you have will increase. But not every day. You will have some off days and some amazing days, but the science and practice in this book will help you trend upward toward six or more high-value experiences every day. This should encourage you to keep doing the prosocial exercises in this book.

Increasing your happiness requires practice because, perhaps surprisingly, your brain is a very lazy organ. It burns about 20 percent of the calories you take in but constitutes only 3 percent of body weight. The body manages this high overhead cost by establishing default pathways in the brain that activate when we encounter similar circumstances. These manifest as habits. For example, when my children were young, I always kept pretzels in the car for snacks. At some point, I realized that every time I got in the car by myself, I would automatically eat pretzels, even if I were not hungry, because I had created the habit of eating pretzels while driving. I had to get rid of the pretzels to rewrite the default neural activation that linked driving to eating pretzels in order to break this habit. Practicing prosocial behaviors using the exercises in this book will do the same thing: you will toss out those stale-pretzel selfish habits and replace them with virtuous prosocial habits that will bring you and those around you moments of joy. Do this consistently and your brain will adapt to being virtuous more often, improving not only your happiness, but your immune system, your sleep, and the motivation to exercise.

How do I know this? In 2010, *Fast Company* magazine ran a feature article after interviewing me and visiting my lab, giving me the nickname "Dr. Love." This came about because my research group has made fundamental insights into the brain basis for happiness, health, and longevity. All of these are improved when we give and receive love. My lab's research has continued since then, ultimately resulting in the development of the SIX app. Tens of thousands of people are already using the SIX app on their journey to greater happiness. But you need to commit to using SIX every day to measure your progress.

Ben Franklin understood the importance of practice to establish the habit of virtue. He discovered that practicing all virtues simultaneously was too hard. Instead, Franklin would practice one virtue each week, "leaving all others to their ordinary chance." This book is similarly structured, giving you one virtue to work on at a time and a box to check when you have practiced each one three times. I expect that this book will be your companion for the next year since it may take a week or so to complete each set of practices.

Each chapter of this book defines one virtue, describes what it does in the brain, and provides practices based on scientific research so you can become a virtue virtuoso. There is a blank page next to each virtue so that you can take notes and build a library of insights on what you learned from your practice.

All the virtues are equally important, so they are presented in alphabetical order. But that is just for convenience. You can read the book and practice the virtues in any order you want. But you must practice to get your lazy, lazy brain to establish new pathways leading to stronger and richer social connections. By his own admission, Franklin failed to behave virtuously many times, and so will you. But he also thought just trying to be virtuous improved his happiness. So please continue to practice the exercises herein.

You are embarking on a journey to improve your life, and there will be times when you just cannot do the exercises in this book. It is fine to take a break and also to return to previous chapters to brush up on virtues you may not have mastered. Or, virtues you just enjoy and want to revisit.

Franklin devoted more pages in his autobiography to discussing the virtues than any other topic in his long and very interesting life. Franklin wrote, "I hope, therefore, that some of my descendants may follow the example and reap the benefit." We can be the intellectual descendants of Benjamin Franklin. The science and practice of the virtues in this little book are just what Franklin would have wanted his intellectual heirs to practice.

1.

ADAPTABILITY

Flexibility in behavior and thinking applied to new situations or information.

SCIENCE

Embracing the new activates dopamine release in the midbrain, facilitating a desire to explore.

INSIGHT

"Enjoying success requires the ability to adapt. Only by being open to change will you have a true opportunity to get the most from your talent."

—NOLAN RYAN, HALL OF FAME PITCHER

PRACTICE

1. Embrace making mistakes by trying a fun or silly activity (bowling, ping-pong, etc.) and getting feedback from someone better than you.
2. Write down everything you learned when something you tried did not go as planned; what can you do differently when you are in a similar situation?
3. Read a nonfiction book on a topic you know little about and write down one way to use what you learned.

DATE COMPLETED AND NOTES

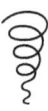

1. ....
   ....
   ....
   ....

2. ....
   ....
   ....
   ....

3. ....
   ....
   ....
   ....

2.
ATTENTION

Full immersion in the present experience.

SCIENCE

Activation of the brain's prefrontal cortex generates conscious attention to an experience and requires sustained effort.

INSIGHT

"The first rule of focus is this: 'Wherever you are, be there.'"
—UNKNOWN

PRACTICE

1. Practice mindfulness meditation using an app for at least one week.
2. Walk in nature and try to identify the species of everything you see (bushes, trees, animals).
3. Read a book for one hour for seven days in a row without other technology interrupting you. (You are doing this now!)

DATE COMPLETED AND NOTES

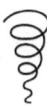

1. ....

   ....

   ....

   ....

2. ....

   ....

   ....

   ....

3. ....

   ....

   ....

   ....

3.

AWE

An overwhelming experience of the extraordinary.

SCIENCE

Awe activates a region in the temporal lobe associated with changing one's frame of reference.

INSIGHT

"The most beautiful thing we can experience is the mysterious."
—ALBERT EINSTEIN, NOBEL LAUREATE PHYSICIST

PRACTICE

1. Climb a hill in the early morning and watch the sun rise.
2. Sit in a holy building when there is no service and absorb the architecture, sounds, and smells.
3. Attend a live concert of elevating music by Bach, Segovia, or another composer; bring a friend to increase its impact.

DATE COMPLETED AND NOTES

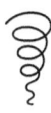

1. ....

   ....

   ....

   ....

2. ....

   ....

   ....

   ....

3. ....

   ....

   ....

   ....

4.

CAUTION

Awareness such that one avoids mistakes or danger.

SCIENCE

The brain's cingulate cortex identifies anomalies in one's environment in half a second and produces bodily sensations such as sweat and "butterflies" in the stomach that should not be ignored.

INSIGHT

"More firm the hand of courage strikes, when it obeys the watchful eye of caution."

—JAMES THOMSON, SCOTTISH POET

PRACTICE

1. Do a "pre-mortem" by writing down three worst-case outcomes before embarking on something new.
2. Delay important decisions by a day to enable the brain to consolidate information during sleep.
3. Seek advice from trusted friends when you are considering a new venture.

DATE COMPLETED AND NOTES

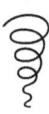

1. ....
   ....
   ....
   ....

2. ....
   ....
   ....
   ....

3. ....
   ....
   ....
   ....

5.

COMPASSION

Awareness of others' distress and a desire to alleviate it.

SCIENCE

Sharing another's distress induces the brain to release oxytocin, which increases empathy and motivates a desire to help.

INSIGHT

"The purpose of human life is to serve, and to show compassion and the will to help others."
—ALBERT SCHWEITZER, NOBEL PEACE PRIZE RECIPIENT

PRACTICE

1. Practice loving-kindness meditation every day for one week using an app where you focus for ten minutes on showing love to those around you, even those you dislike.
2. Write a letter to yourself taking the perspective of someone with whom your relationship is strained or broken.
3. Train being compassionate by doing a small act of kindness for a stranger daily for one week; every day it will become easier.

DATE COMPLETED AND NOTES

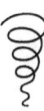

1. ....

   ....

   ....

   ....

2. ....

   ....

   ....

   ....

3. ....

   ....

   ....

   ....

6.

COURAGE

Determination in the face of fear or difficulty.

SCIENCE

The brain can reduce the fear of a difficult activity through the release of endorphins allowing one to do something that seems impossible.

INSIGHT

"Life shrinks or expands in proportion to one's courage."
—ANAÏS NIN, FRENCH-AMERICAN WRITER

PRACTICE

1. Sign up to be instructed in a challenging new activity with a bit of danger that you would not ordinarily do, for example, rock climbing or surfing.
2. Knock on the door of a neighbor you do not know and introduce yourself.
3. If you are healthy enough, fast for one day only consuming liquids during daylight and a broth and electrolytes at night.

DATE COMPLETED AND NOTES

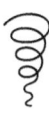

1. ....
....
....
....

2. ....
....
....
....

3. ....
....
....
....

7.

CREATIVITY

Divergent thinking that produces something new and unexpected.

SCIENCE

Decreased activity of executive regions of the brain during daydreaming enables the emergence of creative ideas in the parietal cortex, a brain region enlarged in Albert Einstein.

INSIGHT

"Creativity is allowing yourself to make mistakes. Art is knowing which ones to keep."
—SCOTT ADAMS, AMERICAN CARTOONIST AND WRITER

PRACTICE

1. Write a haiku every day for a week.
2. Follow Ben Franklin and form a "junto" with other creative people and meet monthly to share ideas; follow Ben and do this in a pub.
3. Walk fifteen minutes a day for one week in a quiet place and write down ideas that come to you.

DATE COMPLETED AND NOTES

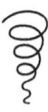

1. ....
   ....
   ....
   ....

2. ....
   ....
   ....
   ....

3. ....
   ....
   ....
   ....

8.

CURIOSITY

Active pursuit of new knowledge and experiences.

SCIENCE

Rich life experiences increase the ability of the brain to discover the new.

INSIGHT

"Curiosity is lying in wait for every secret."
—RALPH WALDO EMERSON, AMERICAN WRITER

PRACTICE

1. Travel to someplace odd in an unfamiliar area, for example, an island or another relatively isolated place, and explore it.
2. Reserve one hour a day on your calendar for a week to explore something or someplace new.
3. Take an online course about something you are curious about and do the homework to earn the certificate of completion.

DATE COMPLETED AND NOTES

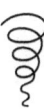

1. ....

   ....

   ....

   ....

2. ....

   ....

   ....

   ....

3. ....

   ....

   ....

   ....

9.
DEFIANCE

Resisting oppressive forces with boldness.

SCIENCE

The prefrontal cortex can suppress neural signals for social or physical discomfort; this is strengthened with practice.

INSIGHT

"I believe ideas matter; the good ones deserve reverence, and the bad ones, defiance."

—NANCY GIBBS, AMERICAN JOURNALIST

PRACTICE

1. For one week, extend by one any activity you do consistently, for example, by walking one more mile or writing for one more hour.
2. Ask a question to a person with whom you disagree using the word "bullshit" to challenge him or her to explain something more clearly.
3. Say no to something you have been asked to do but that you prefer not to do.

DATE COMPLETED AND NOTES

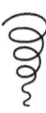

1. ....

....

....

....

2. ....

....

....

....

3. ....

....

....

....

10.

DEVOTION

Ardent dedication to a person or ideal.

SCIENCE

Devotion is encoded in the brain's social-emotional valuation network that sustains consistent attachment.

INSIGHT

"True strength lies in submission which permits one to dedicate his life, through devotion, to something beyond himself."
—HENRY MILLER, AMERICAN WRITER

PRACTICE

1. Make a public commitment or re-commitment to a person you love.
2. Write about your devotion to an ideal, for example, religion or freedom; be brave and post it online.
3. List the ten items you spend the most time on every week; identify a single one that needs your devotion and commit to it.

DATE COMPLETED AND NOTES

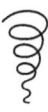

1. ....
   ....
   ....
   ....

2. ....
   ....
   ....
   ....

3. ....
   ....
   ....
   ....

11.

FAIRNESS

Impartiality in thought and action.

SCIENCE

Unfairness activates a brain region that induces a feeling of disgust and reminds us that this is maladaptive.

INSIGHT

"Fair and softly goes far."
—MIGUEL DE CERVANTES, SPANISH WRITER

PRACTICE

1. Write a constitution for an organization you are in, for example, a classroom, work group, or family, asking others to agree on the rules of behavior. Post it prominently.
2. Resolve a dispute using the "Pareto principle": maximize happiness for the group without making anyone worse off.
3. Practice procedural justice by creating a written dispute resolution process that is publicly shared and that everyone agrees to follow.

DATE COMPLETED AND NOTES

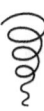

1. ....

   ....

   ....

   ....

2. ....

   ....

   ....

   ....

3. ....

   ....

   ....

   ....

12.
FORGIVENESS

Surrendering resentment and a claim for recompense from another.

SCIENCE
Revenge causes chronic stress and inhibits immune responses; forgiveness eliminates these effects.

INSIGHT
"The weak can never forgive. Forgiveness is the attribute of the strong."
—MAHATMA GANDHI, INDIAN INDEPENDENCE LEADER

PRACTICE
1. Write a letter or email to someone who has wronged you and tell them you forgive them.
2. Every night for a week before you go to sleep, pray or think positive thoughts about someone who has hurt you.
3. Write yourself a letter and forgive yourself for something that has bothered you for a long time; save the letter to reread when needed.

DATE COMPLETED AND NOTES

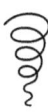

1. ....

   ....

   ....

   ....

2. ....

   ....

   ....

   ....

3. ....

   ....

   ....

   ....

13.

GENEROSITY

Giving freely and abundantly.

SCIENCE

Generosity occurs readily when we share the emotional state of another.

INSIGHT

"Generosity is the most natural outward expression of an inner attitude of compassion and loving-kindness."

—TENZIN GYATSO, 14TH DALAI LAMA

PRACTICE

1. The next time you eat out, double your typical tip and leave before the server receives it.
2. Pay the toll for the person behind you on a road or bridge.
3. Give a gift to a friend or coworker for no occasion at all, telling them why they are special.

DATE COMPLETED AND NOTES

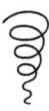

1. ....

   ....

   ....

   ....

2. ....

   ....

   ....

   ....

3. ....

   ....

   ....

   ....

14.

GRATITUDE

A genuine appreciation of another's kindness.

SCIENCE

Brain regions that enable the appreciation of another require focus without distraction.

INSIGHT

"Gratitude is not only the greatest of virtues, but the parent of all the others."

—MARCUS TULLIUS CICERO, ROMAN STATESMAN AND PHILOSOPHER

PRACTICE

1. Every day for one week, tell a person you work with why you are grateful for them as a human being.
2. Keep a gratitude journal: for one month, every night before going to sleep write down three things you were grateful for that day. Assess your happiness at the end of the month.
3. Every day for one week, take a walk and breathe in deeply to smell the environment; try to identify why this makes you happy.

DATE COMPLETED AND NOTES

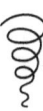

1. ....

   ....

   ....

   ....

2. ....

   ....

   ....

   ....

3. ....

   ....

   ....

   ....

15.

HONESTY

Being truthful, sincere, and transparent.

SCIENCE

Honesty uses fewer cognitive resources than lying, freeing neural bandwidth to foster stronger relationships.

INSIGHT

"Honesty is the first chapter in the book of wisdom."
—THOMAS JEFFERSON, FOUNDING FATHER AND THIRD PRESIDENT OF THE UNITED STATES

PRACTICE

1. Think of a lie you have told to another person and write down why this is damaging to your relationship.
2. Spend an entire day being honest with everyone you encounter (only white lies are allowed if honesty would be hurtful); reflect on how it feels.
3. Repair dishonesty by contacting someone you have lied to and fessing up; you cannot use the word "because" as a justification.

DATE COMPLETED AND NOTES

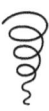

1. ....

   ....

   ....

   ....

2. ....

   ....

   ....

   ....

3. ....

   ....

   ....

   ....

16.
HUMOR

Delighting in the odd, ludicrous, or absurd.

SCIENCE

Humor is intrinsically rewarding to the brain and strengthens relationships when shared with others.

INSIGHT

"Laughter is an instant vacation."
—MILTON BERLE, AMERICAN COMEDIAN

PRACTICE

1. Start funny hat day or ugly sweater day with your work colleagues on Fridays.
2. Attend a live comedy show with a friend.
3. Buy a joke-a-day calendar or sign up for a joke sent by email so you smile in the morning.

DATE COMPLETED AND NOTES

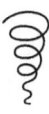

1. ....
   ....
   ....
   ....

2. ....
   ....
   ....
   ....

3. ....
   ....
   ....
   ....

17.
IMPARTIALITY

Treating every person and situation without bias, even when you have a stake in the outcome.

SCIENCE

Fair treatment is more likely to occur when decision rules are decided in advance and written down.

INSIGHT

"It is wisest to be impartial."
—PARAMAHANSA YOGANANDA, INDIAN YOGI

PRACTICE

1. Count to five before making a decision, suppressing your immediate reaction and giving yourself time to assess what is fair.
2. During your next disagreement, switch roles and argue in favor of the other person's view and have them do the same for you.
3. Crowdsource a consequential decision by sharing the pros and cons with five or more friends, asking them to vote, and making the vote binding.

DATE COMPLETED AND NOTES

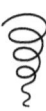

1. ....

....

....

....

2. ....

....

....

....

3. ....

....

....

....

18.

INDUSTRIOUSNESS

Applying oneself consistently and energetically.

SCIENCE

Feedback between the brain's prefrontal cortex, which sustains focus, and regions that process rewarding behaviors that support industriousness can be strengthened with practice.

INSIGHT

"I was obliged to be industrious. Whoever is equally industrious will succeed equally well."
—JOHANN SEBASTIAN BACH, GERMAN COMPOSER

PRACTICE

1. Use a calendar to block out time for specific tasks so you are not interrupted and can complete them.
2. For one week, wake up daily at 5 a.m. and assess if you get more done.
3. Use a daily list of tasks in which you order the list by importance, and enjoy the satisfaction of checking tasks off when done.

DATE COMPLETED AND NOTES

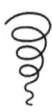

1. ....
   ....
   ....
   ....

2. ....
   ....
   ....
   ....

3. ....
   ....
   ....
   ....

19.

INNOCENCE

Arriving in situations with openness and optimism.

SCIENCE

The brain can be "reset" toward innocence by inhibiting one's internal dialog to focus on the present experience.

INSIGHT

"I might have some character traits that some might see as innocence or naive. That's because I discovered peace and happiness in my soul. And with this knowledge, I also see the beauty of human life."

—TOBEY MAGUIRE, AMERICAN ACTOR

PRACTICE

1. In your next meeting, empower others to share by saying, "Help me understand this."
2. Avoid disparaging people psychologically by presuming everyone has good intentions, especially difficult people.
3. Spend two weeks re-learning a subject that you dislike, but do so without negative emotions; engage an instructor to help you if you want to make it easier.

DATE COMPLETED AND NOTES

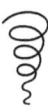

1. ....

   ....

   ....

   ....

2. ....

   ....

   ....

   ....

3. ....

   ....

   ....

   ....

20.
JUSTICE

Treating others as you would want them to treat you.

SCIENCE

Frontal brain regions associated with cognitive control enable people to be just.

INSIGHT

"If you want peace, work for justice."
—GIOVANNI MONTINI, POPE PAUL VI

PRACTICE

1. Recall a recent time that you were treated unjustly and write down how your future self would react to this ten years from now.
2. Ensure justice is not self-serving by asking a trusted friend how to deal with a difficult person or problem.
3. When making a decision that impacts another person, write down pros and cons for the other person to gain their perspective.

DATE COMPLETED AND NOTES

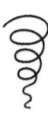

1. ....

   ....

   ....

   ....

2. ....

   ....

   ....

   ....

3. ....

   ....

   ....

   ....

21.

LOVE

The strong emotional desire to put another's needs before one's own.

SCIENCE

The neurochemicals of attachment, especially oxytocin and dopamine, synchronize emotional states with those we love.

INSIGHT

"Being deeply loved by someone gives you strength, while loving someone deeply gives you courage."

—LAO TZU, CHINESE PHILOSOPHER

PRACTICE

1. Use the Love+ algorithm: try to add love into the world with every interaction you have.
2. Every day for a week, give at least eight people a hug.
3. For seven days in a row, tell one nonfamily member that you love them.

DATE COMPLETED AND NOTES

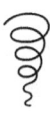

1. ....
   ....
   ....
   ....

2. ....
   ....
   ....
   ....

3. ....
   ....
   ....
   ....

22.

LOYALTY

Commitment to a person or cause.

SCIENCE

Loyalty requires both cognitive commitment, and emotional attachment that often occurs after an extraordinary experience.

INSIGHT

"I have a loyalty that runs in my bloodstream, when I lock into someone or something, you can't get me away from it because I commit that thoroughly. That's in friendship, that's a deal, that's a commitment. Don't give me paper—I can get the same lawyer who drew it up to break it. But if you shake my hand, that's for life."
—JERRY LEWIS, AMERICAN COMEDIAN AND ACTOR

PRACTICE

1. For seven days in a row, perform an unexpected task to help another person, for example, bring food, bring coffee, or pick up a task they typically do.
2. Make a pledge to a family member that you will be of service to them for whatever they need and whenever they need it and see how they react.
3. Establish a sheepdog mindset: be responsible for those around you by looking after their interests; practice this by helping two strangers today.

DATE COMPLETED AND NOTES

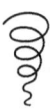

1. ....

   ....

   ....

   ....

2. ....

   ....

   ....

   ....

3. ....

   ....

   ....

   ....

23.
MAJESTY

Behaving with dignity and grace.

SCIENCE

Majesty requires being acutely aware of how one's behaviors influence the emotional responses of others.

INSIGHT

"There is a certain majesty in simplicity which is far above all the quaintness of wit."

—ALEXANDER POPE, BRITISH POET

PRACTICE

1. The next three times you eat at a restaurant, show respect to those serving you by calling them sir and ma'am and see how they respond.
2. Introduce yourself to sales staff when shopping using your first name, and address the person helping you by their first name.
3. The next time you attend a meeting, dress sharply to show others that the occasion is important.

DATE COMPLETED AND NOTES

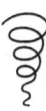

1. ....

   ....

   ....

   ....

2. ....

   ....

   ....

   ....

3. ....

   ....

   ....

   ....

24.

MODERATION

Choosing to remain within reasonable limits.

SCIENCE

Slowing down decisions increases the ability to moderate choices by inhibiting impulsive desires.

INSIGHT

"Moderation in temper is always a virtue; but moderation in principle is always a vice."
—THOMAS PAINE, PATRIOT OF THE AMERICAN REVOLUTION

PRACTICE

1. For one week, get up early and walk for at least twenty minutes.
2. Forgo dessert after dinner for a week and see how this makes you feel.
3. Abstain from alcohol during Sober October or another month you choose. If you do not drink alcohol, give up another drink you enjoy, such as coffee or tea.

DATE COMPLETED AND NOTES

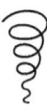

1. ....

   ....

   ....

   ....

2. ....

   ....

   ....

   ....

3. ....

   ....

   ....

   ....

25.

MODESTY

Freedom from conceit or vanity.

SCIENCE

Actively focus on being a less important person by cultivating a genuine interest in the welfare of others.

INSIGHT

"Modesty is the conscience of the body."
—HONORÉ DE BALZAC, FRENCH NOVELIST AND PLAYWRIGHT

PRACTICE

1. Take a friend to lunch and do not use the word "I" for thirty minutes.
2. At your next meeting, see how long you can keep quiet even if you are in charge.
3. Institute an AMA ("ask me anything") monthly for colleagues, friends, or family and answer questions honestly.

DATE COMPLETED AND NOTES

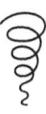

1. ....

....

....

....

2. ....

....

....

....

3. ....

....

....

....

26.

OBEDIENCE

Thoughtfully deferring to another's wishes.

SCIENCE

A brain region called the temporal-parietal junction enables us to take another's perspective and can be activated through physical mimicry.

INSIGHT

"Better than worshiping gods is obedience to the laws of righteousness."

—SIDDHARTHA GAUTAMA, THE BUDDHA

PRACTICE

1. Ask your romantic partner or roommate what chores they would like you to do for a week.
2. Empower someone you work with to make an important decision, even if you disagree with it.
3. Hire a personal trainer or nutritionist for five sessions and strictly follow the recommended workout or diet.

DATE COMPLETED AND NOTES

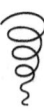

1. ....

....

....

....

2. ....

....

....

....

3. ....

....

....

....

27.

OPENNESS

A desire for new ideas and experiences.

SCIENCE

The brain's default mode network stimulates creativity, which becomes active when external stimulation is absent.

INSIGHT

"Creativity has always depended on openness and flexibility."
—SIRI HUSTVEDT, AMERICAN NOVELIST

PRACTICE

1. Ask a friend to suggest a book that you probably will not like. Read it.
2. For one week, listen to a podcast that supports the opposite view of an opinion you hold.
3. Ask a friend to organize a trip that you will join without asking you for any input.

DATE COMPLETED AND NOTES

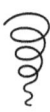

1. ....
   ....
   ....
   ....

2. ....
   ....
   ....
   ....

3. ....
   ....
   ....
   ....

28.

PATIENCE

Bearing annoyance without complaining.

SCIENCE

Concentrated activity in the brain's prefrontal cortex enables patience by deferring the desire for immediate gratification.

INSIGHT

"You must first have a lot of patience to learn to have patience."
—STANISLAW JERZY LEC, POLISH POET

PRACTICE

1. Put a sign that says "Patience" on your car dashboard for a month as a reminder to drive carefully.
2. For one day, be conscious not to interrupt anyone, especially subordinates, by counting 1-2-3 before speaking.
3. Spend one hour visiting an elderly friend or family member whose stories you already know well and let them talk.

DATE COMPLETED AND NOTES

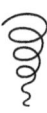

1. ....

   ....

   ....

   ....

2. ....

   ....

   ....

   ....

3. ....

   ....

   ....

   ....

29.

PATRIOTISM

Devotion to one's country.

SCIENCE

Patriotism is an emotional attachment that results in joy when viewing national symbols and outrage when national norms are violated.

INSIGHT

"Patriotism must be founded on great principles and supported by great virtue."

—KING HENRY IV OF ENGLAND

PRACTICE

1. Fly your country's flag in front of your house for a month and see what kinds of conversations happen with your neighbors.
2. Wear a shirt with your country's flag on it and discuss with others why you are patriotic.
3. Volunteer at a local veterans event or medical center and talk to members about their military service.

DATE COMPLETED AND NOTES

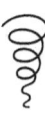

1. ....

....

....

....

2. ....

....

....

....

3. ....

....

....

....

30.

PERSEVERANCE

Bearing difficulties calmly and without complaint.

SCIENCE

Practicing sustained performance in one task can make perseverance in other tasks easier.

INSIGHT

"Perseverance is not a long race; it is many short races one after the other."

—WALTER ELLIOT, SCOTTISH POLITICIAN

PRACTICE

1. If you are healthy enough, increase your exercise by 50 percent for a day; reflect on how you feel.
2. Finish the long book on your nightstand or buy a thick book and read it.
3. Eat vegetarian for one week. (If you are a vegetarian, do number 1 or 2 twice.)

DATE COMPLETED AND NOTES

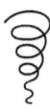

1. ....

....

....

....

2. ....

....

....

....

3. ....

....

....

....

31.

PRUDENCE

Being deliberate and careful in one's choices.

SCIENCE

Choosing a moral exemplar and following what they do helps establish prudent behaviors.

INSIGHT

"In matters of conscience, first thoughts are best. In matters of prudence, last thoughts are best."

—ROBERT HALL, ENGLISH CLERGYMAN

PRACTICE

1. Delay purchasing items online for twenty-four hours to ensure you really need them; do this for a week by putting a sign on your computer.
2. Do not purchase any new clothes for yourself for six months.
3. Set up an automatic monthly transfer of 10 percent of your salary to a no-load mutual fund to learn to live on less and fund your retirement.

DATE COMPLETED AND NOTES

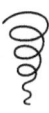

1. ....

   ....

   ....

   ....

2. ....

   ....

   ....

   ....

3. ....

   ....

   ....

   ....

32.

PURPOSE

Acting deliberately to accomplish the most important objectives of your life.

SCIENCE

Purpose is discovered and sustained when an activity produces a feeling of joy.

INSIGHT

"True happiness...is not attained through self-gratification, but through fidelity to a worthy purpose."

—HELEN KELLER, AMERICAN AUTHOR AND DISABILITY RIGHTS ADVOCATE

PRACTICE

1. Over the course of a week, write down ideas for your purpose in life until you converge on the best answer.
2. Send your purpose statement to three friends to get their feedback, and ask them about their purposes.
3. Make a list of things you can do to live your purpose and do at least one of them within a month.

DATE COMPLETED AND NOTES

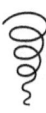

1. ....

   ....

   ....

   ....

2. ....

   ....

   ....

   ....

3. ....

   ....

   ....

   ....

33.
RESPONSIBILITY

Being reliable in words and deeds.

SCIENCE
Following established rules or norms of behavior makes decisions easier and faster.

INSIGHT
"The price of greatness is responsibility."
—WINSTON CHURCHILL, BRITISH STATESMAN AND WRITER

PRACTICE
1. For one week, drive exactly the speed limit and reflect how it made you feel.
2. Rank ten things you are responsible for this week and eliminate the bottom five so you can focus on the others.
3. Write down three times you were irresponsible; diagnose why you behaved this way.

DATE COMPLETED AND NOTES

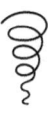

1. ....

   ....

   ....

   ....

2. ....

   ....

   ....

   ....

3. ....

   ....

   ....

   ....

34.

SELF-REGULATION

Maintaining equanimity in difficult circumstances.

SCIENCE

You can improve self-regulation during stress by taking deep breaths and holding them for five seconds before exhaling.

INSIGHT

"Self-regulation depends on having a friendly relationship with your body. Without it you have to rely on external regulation—from medication, drugs like alcohol, constant reassurance, or compulsive compliance with the wishes of others."

—BESSEL A. VAN DER KOLK, DUTCH PSYCHIATRIST AND AUTHOR

PRACTICE

1. Rewatch a movie that made you cry and focus on not crying.
2. Make a commitment to a friend to call each other when either of you is upset to regulate emotional states.
3. Write down three presumed reasons that a person in your life is abrasive and recall these reasons when you interact with them.

DATE COMPLETED AND NOTES

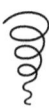

1. ....
   ....
   ....
   ....

2. ....
   ....
   ....
   ....

3. ....
   ....
   ....
   ....

35.

SENSITIVITY

Awareness of the needs and emotions of others.

SCIENCE

Understanding others requires focusing on others' needs rather than our own to enable empathy.

INSIGHT

"Ultimately, my character is defined by the quality of my sensitivity to other people. I exist in equilibrium. I am here to the degree I am there."

—HUGH PRATHER, AMERICAN WRITER

PRACTICE

1. Listen with your eyes; look at the face of a person with whom you are talking rather than somewhere else.
2. Create an "electronics Shabbat"; pick one day a week when your entire household does not use any electronic devices in order to connect more deeply with each other.
3. When talking to a romantic partner or friend, tell them you will ask them "why" five times to fully understand the topic they are sharing.

DATE COMPLETED AND NOTES

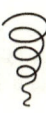

1. ....

2. ....

3. ....

36.

SERENITY

Maintaining internal calmness and acceptance.

SCIENCE

Serenity is actively evaluative, rather than passively observational, generating an understanding of the essence of an experience.

INSIGHT

"Boredom is the feeling that everything is a waste of time; serenity, that nothing is."
—THOMAS SZASZ, HUNGARIAN-AMERICAN PSYCHIATRIST

PRACTICE

1. Create a short mantra that is meaningful to you and say it for three minutes every hour on the hour for a week.
2. Take a walk at half your normal pace and concentrate on feeling all five of your senses.
3. Identify a person who causes friction and say to yourself "accept" while they speak.

DATE COMPLETED AND NOTES

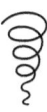

1. ....
   ....
   ....
   ....

2. ....
   ....
   ....
   ....

3. ....
   ....
   ....
   ....

37.

SILENCE

The absence of internal or external stimulation.

SCIENCE

Silence enables the brain's default mode network to generate spontaneous cognition that manifests as flashes of insight.

INSIGHT

"Everything that's created comes out of silence. Your thoughts emerge from the nothingness of silence. Your words come out of this void. Your very essence emerged from emptiness. All creativity requires some stillness."
—WAYNE DYER, AMERICAN SELF-DEVELOPMENT WRITER

PRACTICE

1. Sit in a comfortable position in silence for twenty minutes first thing in the morning for a week; reflect on what you thought about.
2. For one week, block out two hours every day for silent work and evaluate your productivity; use noise-canceling headphones if your space is noisy.
3. Find a forest or nature preserve in which you can walk for one hour without headphones; share a photo of the most interesting thing you see with a friend to start a conversation about silence.

DATE COMPLETED AND NOTES

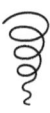

1. ....

   ....

   ....

   ....

2. ....

   ....

   ....

   ....

3. ....

   ....

   ....

   ....

38.

SINCERITY

Being free from pretense and avoiding deceit.

SCIENCE

Insincerity induces physiologic stress that drains one's energy and is unconsciously perceived by others, damaging relationships.

INSIGHT

"Sincerity may be humble but she cannot be servile."
—LORD BYRON, ENGLISH ROMANTIC POET

PRACTICE

1. When asked your opinion, give honest feedback but do so kindly if it is negative.
2. Make amends for insincerity: email three people to whom you have been insincere and offer them an apology.
3. Ask three family members or friends to honestly complete this sentence about you: "You are genuinely sincere when you _____." Ask them why they believe this.

DATE COMPLETED AND NOTES

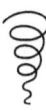

1. ....

   ....

   ....

   ....

2. ....

   ....

   ....

   ....

3. ....

   ....

   ....

   ....

39.

SPONTANEITY

Responding to the present moment without restraint.

SCIENCE

Spontaneity is inhibited by over-analyzing a situation; responding with your first impulse results in spontaneous actions.

INSIGHT

"Only in spontaneity can we be who we truly are."
—JOHN MCLAUGHLIN, ENGLISH MUSICIAN

PRACTICE

1. Ask a friend to join you someplace fun but without a plan of what to do.
2. Ask a friend to choose a day trip for you and go there by yourself.
3. For one week, say "yes" to anything someone asks you to do.

DATE COMPLETED AND NOTES

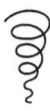

1. ....

   ....

   ....

   ....

2. ....

   ....

   ....

   ....

3. ....

   ....

   ....

   ....

40.

TEAMWORK

Contributing effort to further others' goals.

SCIENCE

Teamwork is more effective when you understand why something is important to others and when you know them well.

INSIGHT

"Teamwork is what the Green Bay Packers were all about. They didn't do it for individual glory. They did it because they loved one another."

—VINCE LOMBARDI, LEADING AMERICAN FOOTBALL COACH

PRACTICE

1. Volunteer to do the most difficult or dirty part of a task at work or home every day for a week.
2. Surprise your team or family with a celebration when they reach a meaningful milestone.
3. In your next team meeting, ask each member to offer one example of how their work improves people's lives.

DATE COMPLETED AND NOTES

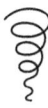

1. ....
   ....
   ....
   ....

2. ....
   ....
   ....
   ....

3. ....
   ....
   ....
   ....

41.

TOLERANCE

Accepting and validating others' individuality.

SCIENCE

The human brain has a region devoted to understanding others' motivations. This region is slower to activate than are emotional responses but facilitates accepting people as they are.

INSIGHT

"In the practice of tolerance, one's enemy is the best teacher."
—TENZIN GYATSO, FOURTEENTH DALAI LAMA

PRACTICE

1. The next time you have a difference of opinion on a topic you care about, ask the other person to explain their view rather than defending your position.
2. Create an "opposite day" where you do the opposite of what you normally do; you can start by greeting people with "heaven up" (the opposite of "hel(l)-low").
3. Attend a parade or other celebration, without judgment, for a group that you typically avoid; afterward, call a friend and share your impressions.

DATE COMPLETED AND NOTES

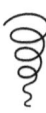

1. ....

   ....

   ....

   ....

2. ....

   ....

   ....

   ....

3. ....

   ....

   ....

   ....

42.

TOUGHNESS

Uncompromising determination when facing obstacles.

SCIENCE

Toughness is built in small steps that train the brain to accept uncomfortableness.

INSIGHT

"We are what we repeatedly do. Excellence, therefore, is not an act but a habit."

—ARISTOTLE, GREEK PHILOSOPHER

PRACTICE

1. Delay your midday meal by one hour for seven straight days.
2. Try a cold plunge and see how you feel.
3. Face a fear by intentionally exposing yourself to it safely, for example, visit the snake exhibit at a zoo, go tandem skydiving, or visit a country where you do not speak the language.

DATE COMPLETED AND NOTES

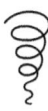

1. ....

....

....

....

2. ....

....

....

....

3. ....

....

....

....

43.

TRUST

Intentionally relying on another person.

SCIENCE

The absence of a fear signal in the brain motivates trust, especially toward strangers.

INSIGHT

"Love all, trust a few, do wrong to none."
—WILLIAM SHAKESPEARE, ENGLISH PLAYWRIGHT AND POET

PRACTICE

1. Let a child plan a Saturday for you.
2. Ask a romantic partner or friend to make you dinner and eat it blindfolded; see how many foods you can identify by taste and smell alone.
3. Ask a close friend or neighbor to hold the key to your house in case you should ever need them to enter it.

DATE COMPLETED AND NOTES

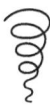

1. ....
   ....
   ....
   ....

2. ....
   ....
   ....
   ....

3. ....
   ....
   ....
   ....

44.

TRUSTWORTHINESS

Reciprocating the confidence someone has placed in you.

SCIENCE

The brain's release of oxytocin is stimulated by any kindness, which, in turn, motivates trustworthiness.

INSIGHT

"No virtue is more universally accepted as a test of good character than trustworthiness."

—HARRY EMERSON FOSDICK, AMERICAN PASTOR

PRACTICE

1. Tell two people you are their "3 a.m. friend," meaning they can depend on you to be there for them no matter what, even at 3 a.m.
2. Write down a description of a situation when you were not trustworthy; try to identify an explanation for your failing.
3. Offer to babysit or pet sit for a neighbor so they can have a night out or get away for a weekend.

DATE COMPLETED AND NOTES

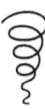

1. ....

....

....

....

2. ....

....

....

....

3. ....

....

....

....

45.

WISDOM

Contextualizing knowledge, leading to good judgment.

SCIENCE

The brain's association cortices, which require decades to acquire sufficient information, build models of the world that result in wisdom.

INSIGHT

"By three methods we may learn wisdom: First, by reflection, which is noblest; Second, by imitation, which is easiest; and third by experience, which is the bitterest."
—CONFUCIUS, CHINESE PHILOSOPHER

PRACTICE

1. Interview someone who is eighty years old or older and ask them what wisdom they have acquired.
2. Make a "do not do" list of things you will give up to have the neural bandwidth to gain wisdom.
3. Write down the five most important things you have learned in life so far; discuss this with a group of friends to receive feedback.

DATE COMPLETED AND NOTES

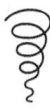

1. ....

   ....

   ....

   ....

2. ....

   ....

   ....

   ....

3. ....

   ....

   ....

   ....

CONCLUSION

Congratulations! You have done something extraordinary and deserve praise. You are now the intellectual child of Benjamin Franklin and can virtuously and humbly share what you have learned with your junto. We should remember that Franklin was a virtuous wild man. He was sexually active, enjoyed food and drink, and was incessantly curious about everything and everyone. It was his energy, tempered by virtue, that drew people toward him.

By some accounts Franklin slept through much of the Continental Congress that rancorously argued how the thirteen American colonies should separate from their British overlords. But when he spoke, he spoke humbly and with insight gained from his expansive experiences and joy for life. Franklin was beloved in life and mourned by nearly all in death.

I expect that you, too, having completed this book, will be beloved by those who know you and by those who meet you for the first time. When I realized and began to practice my purpose in life, to be of service to others, I immediately benefited by sharing the joy of those whom I served. Joy is contagious and it reinforced my own journey toward greater happiness. Of course, I fail like everyone else, and am sometimes less kind toward others than I should be. Yet, I am blessed by the many people who both show me and tell me that they love me every day. I am profoundly privileged to love them back and share the "L" word with as many people I can.

Thank you for taking this journey with Dr. Love. When you add love to the world by serving others, happiness follows. That is the essence of love and the source of a satisfied life. I cannot promise you will live longer when you are virtuous, even though the data shows most people will, but you will live better. This will extend your "playspan," the time you get to play with others in the game of life.

I love you.

www.ingramcontent.com/pod-product-compliance
Lightning Source LLC
Chambersburg PA
CBHW060533080526
44586CB00012B/723